First Degree
Reiki
Manual

First Degree
Reiki
Manual

Eleanor Haspel-Portner, Ph.D.

First Degree Reiki Manual
Eleanor Haspel-Portner, Ph.D.

Copyright © 2023 Noble Sciences, LLC.

ISBN:
978-1-931053-08-2 (Paperback)
978-1-931053-07-5 (Paperback)
978-1-931053-00-6 (Ebook)

Other titles by Eleanor Haspel-Portner
Cosmic Secrets
Patterns of Orientation
Marriage in Trouble: A Time of Decision
Astrology Essentials
Second Degree Reiki Manual & Journal

Author's websites
www.nobleenergywellness.com
www.DrEleanor.com

www.moptu.com/DrEleanor

Illustrations created by Eleanor Haspel-Portner, Ph.D and Cindy Smith
Book Design by Michelle M. White

Important Note:
Material in this manual is not intended to replace a one-on-one relationship with a qualified health care professional. It is not intended as medical advice. This Manual shares knowledge and information based only on the research and experience of the authors. You are advised and encouraged to consult with your health care professional regarding all matters that concern your health.

Your personal health care professionals are important for consultation regarding all matter related to your health. Only your personal health care professional is qualified to recommended to diagnose, treat, cure, and prevent specific medical and psychological problems. Symptoms often require diagnosis or immediate attention. This manual is not a substitution for qualified medical or psychological help for your conditions. Noble Sciences, LLC. strongly advises that the reader seek professional advice before making any health decision. Reiki is not a substitute for medical or psychological treatment.

While all materials and resources are posted in good faith, the accuracy, validity, effectiveness, completeness, or usefulness of any of this information, as with any publication, cannot be guaranteed. Noble Sciences, LLC. accepts no responsibility or liability whatsoever for the use or misuse of the information contained in this manual.

◆ ◆ ◆

Dr. Mikao Usui & Mrs. Hawayo Takata
brought Reiki to us in its pure form.
We carry it with light, love, and integrity
honoring pure tradition.

◆ ◆ ◆

Contents

FOREWORD

1

INTRODUCTION

5

EXPLORING THE DEPTHS OF REIKI

9

THE REIKI TREATMENT
AND HAND POSITIONS

24

CULTIVATING YOUR PRACTICE OF REIKI

55

THE REIKI STORY

59

ABOUT THE AUTHOR

71

COLLABORATIVE ASSISTANCE

73

FOREWORD

Shortly after I began the practice of Transcendental Meditation in January 1974, I began having experiences that I could not explain with my scientific mind. I was already a clinical psychologist and in training as a Jungian Analyst, so when I began having dreams about knowing with a "K", I was open to receiving new awareness. Nevertheless, I was a bit surprised when my first "big" energy experience occurred. At the time, I was sitting quietly when I suddenly experienced a brilliant light coming toward me. I gasped in awe as the light's brilliance surrounded and enveloped me. My awareness opened, activating and expanding my understanding and knowledge of the universe and of consciousness.

Many shifts in my consciousness continued. I remembered seeing auras from the time I was born, and I began to reclaim my psychic gifts while working with clients. Then, during my first trip to the Los Angeles area in August 1976, I recognized that the area around Pacific Palisades was my true home. Shortly thereafter, I decided to relocate my home, family, and private clinical psychology practice there. As I was preparing to move in June 1977, I was told by a colleague to check out a healing modality called Reiki. I took his advice and had the great fortune to attend a First-Degree Reiki class with Mrs. Hawayo Takata, who brought

Reiki from Japan to the western world, in attendance. Thus, I heard Mrs. Takata tell her story and learned directly from her about her experiences using Reiki.

The first night after my first Reiki experience, I treated my head positions using Reiki energy. The following morning, I awoke and immediately noticed that I could see without putting on my glasses. This convinced me that Reiki was a real healing modality, since my myopia was so severe at that time that I could not even see the face of a person standing three feet away from me. So, seeing clearly across a room and seeing street signs at a distance proved to me that something very profound had happened from my Reiki experience and treatment.

As I understand it, Reiki is a white light energy transmitted from Master to student in the "oral" tradition of the past. Reiki initiations are always done in person or at a distance using a formula handed down through generations from master to student. The activation of the energy in a student is done according to a formula that imprints the Reiki symbols and their energy into the student's aura or energy field.

A student, once initiated by a Reiki Master/Teacher, is imprinted with Reiki energy in their auric field for their lifetime. Reiki energy then automatically activates in their hands whenever they touch any living thing, including themselves. No shift in consciousness is required and no additional attunements or initiations are necessary.

After my initial Reiki experiences, I embarked on a journey to integrate Reiki into my other healing modalities in my work and life. I took Second Degree Reiki within a few weeks. And when

Third Degree Reiki was offered after Mrs. Hawayo Takata passed the Reiki keys to her successors, I became the tenth Reiki Master/ Teacher in the West. Reiki has been an integral part of my life and work since I first studied it.

In Loving Light,

Eleanor Haspel-Portner, Ph.D.

Eleanor Haspel-Portner, Ph.D.
Mount Pleasant, South Carolina

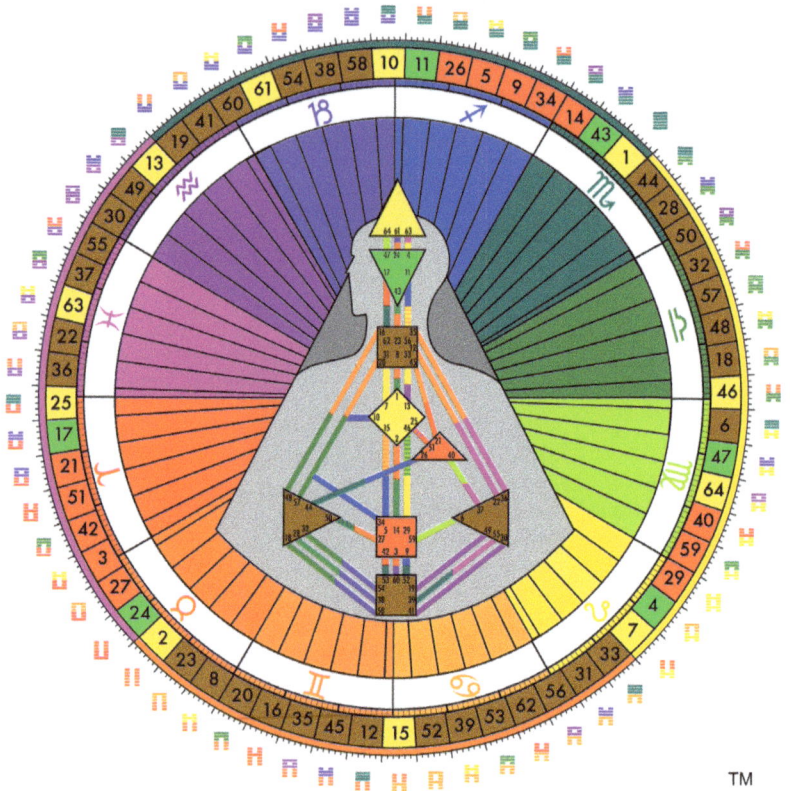

The Mandala of Synthesis – The Integrated World

♦ ♦ ♦

INTRODUCTION

The opportunity to study and utilize Reiki as a tool for healing and wholeness was passed to us through Mrs. Hawayo Takata and then through her successors. When I studied First Degree Reiki, I had the honor of meeting Mrs. Takata and I heard her story directly from her. The following is a brief summary of what she told me.

Her story began when she was a young, widowed woman with two small children. Her health was compromised and she was very weak. She travelled from her home in Hawaii to Japan to have surgery, but she was so frail and ill after the voyage, that she had to wait until she gained enough stamina to withstand the operation. By her description, it took many months in Japan for her to be strong enough for the doctors to agree to do surgery on her.

Finally, the day arrived, and Mrs. Takata was on the operating table. As the team was preparing her for surgery, she heard her deceased husband's voice tell her that "there is another way." This repeated three times. Mrs. Takata described jumping up off the table, much to everyone's chagrin.

She said to the surgeon, "there is another way." He acknowledged that she was right, and he told her about Reiki and said that it would take time.

Mrs. Takata described the difficulties she encountered along her path to becoming a Reiki Master. Part of the difficulty came from the fact that Mrs. Takata was Hawaiian of Japanese ancestry, and Reiki was only given to Japanese citizens. Mrs. Takata's determination paid off, and she was admitted to the program to study Reiki with Dr. Chujiro Hayashi. It took her a year of study in Japan doing Reiki treatments daily. She described riding on trains to visit clients and the difficulty for her because of the circumstances of her life.

Her story was compelling and showed her depth of commitment and her recognition of the powerful healing energy that she was led to bring to the West. Remember, Mrs. Takata was a widow with two young children at this time. After her training was done, she returned to Hawaii.

Mrs. Takata was guided to travel to Japan to be with Dr. Hayashi prior to World War II. He told her about the war and how to protect herself, and he named Mrs. Takata his successor shortly before he died. After the war, all the Reiki Masters in Japan disappeared, leaving Mrs. Takata, who lived in Hawaii, the only living Reiki Master in the World.

At the time I studied Reiki in June of 1977, there were only three Reiki Masters in the West. Anyone could study First Degree Reiki. Students who were interested could ask to study Second Degree Reiki. Third Degree Master/Teacher was by invitation only and was a lifelong commitment.

I completed First Degree, and Second Degree training in July 1977. I immediately had my children initiated into First and Second Degree Reiki. At the time, I had a private practice as a clinical psychologist in Pacific Palisades, California. I used Reiki on my clients regularly. By the time someone walked into my office, I had already done my symbols and was working on them energetically. My clients understood about energy and welcomed the experience of Reiki.

In 1981 we met Barbara Ray who had been given the keys to the Usui Reiki by Mrs. Takata. At the time, Barbara was following the specificity of the attunements to Reiki, and she was honored to be doing the work she was doing.

All my clients and all of Marvin's patients studied Reiki in 1981. In 1982, when Barbara returned to initiate our clients and patients into Second Degree Reiki, we studied and became the tenth and eleventh Reiki Master/Teachers.

Shortly after we became Reiki Master/Teachers, Barbara began initiating Reiki Master/Teachers without vetting them sufficiently. Reiki began to get diluted, and Barbara branched off on her own and developed the Radiance Technique. Phyllis Lei Fukumoto, Mrs. Takata's granddaughter, carried the banner of Usui Shiki Ryoho and founded the Reiki Alliance to preserve the tradition and purity of the real Reiki teaching.

Since Reiki was handed down as an oral tradition with initiations done according to a specific formula and is performed the same way by all Reiki Master/Teachers, it is important that all Master/Teachers honor the teaching intact. Anyone who studies Reiki from a member of the Reiki Alliance can be assured that the teaching carries the pure white light energy so powerful with Reiki.

This manual contains my notes from my First Degree Reiki class when Mrs. Takata was present. Because I studied Reiki with Mrs. Takata, it was emphasized that the Reiki Symbols were sacred energy and that when we drew them on paper, it was important to burn the paper or properly dispose of it because the symbols have energy. In addition, studying Reiki was seen as a sacred trust and those initiated had a responsibility to preserve the teaching intact and exactly as it was taught.

Mrs. Takata shared many of her experiences and information she had gained from her work through the years with Reiki in terms of what each position treats and how the energy moves. This manual presents the notes I took in my First Degree Reiki class because much of what was outlined in my notes came from Mrs. Takata directly. It was my privilege to be in her presence and to learn directly from her. The information in this manual is presented so you can easily reference it while doing a treatment.

Exploring the
Depths of Reiki

FIRST DEGREE REIKI

With the study of First Degree Reiki, the hands become a channel for transmitting pure white light energy upon physical contact with living matter. The experience of First Degree Reiki generally has a profound effect on its students. With no alteration of consciousness through meditation, the healing energies of Reiki flow through the body on contact. No one needs any special attainment of supernatural or mystical powers to learn Reiki.

Students of Reiki, upon receiving the First Degree that activates energy transmissions, become channels of the highest vibration energies known. As channels of healing energies, First Degree students can use Reiki on themselves and on others to facilitate healing on whatever level healing must occur to achieve wholeness.

By its very nature, Reiki energy works naturally toward wholeness. Reiki energy is life force energy or chi. This energy moves in a spiraling formation much as the energy of creation moves in a spiral formation. This pattern of movement flows with life toward health and consciousness, and toward wholeness.

Through the years of my work with Reiki, many students expressed a deepening sense of inspiration and empowerment after being attuned to the different levels of Reiki. While each person experiences Reiki energy in a different way, most people genuinely feel something happening in their hands, on those that they touch, and within themselves. Reiki unlocks a white light healing power that already exists within each of us, connecting us to the Divinity within. In illuminating that force, the white light healing energy connects us more cohesively to our own life force energy. Taken from another perspective, people often feel personal transformation.

As individuals become aware of themselves using or channeling this Reiki healing light, some people experience subtle changes while other people experience dramatic transformation. People are often compelled to practice Reiki and to continue with Second and sometimes Third Degree (Mastery) because it helps them understand aspects of healing light energy. Most people experience Reiki healing light energy and this life force energy as profound.

With Reiki, deepening the understanding that you are more than just a holder of the light enlivens within you. You recognize that you are a conduit and transmitter of light. The more you comprehend this, the more freedom you tend to feel in all aspects of your life. This is why, very often, students remark that they actually feel energized when they do Reiki on others. During Reiki healing, energy passes through you. This energy runs through everyone, joining everyone together as it heals. No personal energy is ever used in Reiki.

SECOND DEGREE REIKI

Second Degree Reiki allows an individual to move beyond the limits of physical space into another dimension of experience. The profound experience of First Degree Reiki becomes magnified and expands with Second Degree Reiki; it becomes activated through a set of energy transmissions. Students become a channel directing white light energy through time and space. Healing can be done at a distance on one or more individuals in the present, past, or future. Second Degree Reiki students often feel stirring excitement much as they did with First Degree Reiki—a sense that a deep knowing is being re-awakened.

In working with consciousness, individuals often experience a deep sense of recognition for those components that draw them to unifying knowledge in its symbolic form. Reiki activates some of the recognition of the energetic components of this knowledge without the mind having to grasp information in an intellectual way. All humans enter an energetic field of unity when they are asleep because at that time their consciousness shifts away from mental analysis and the interpretations it carries, and away from the field of human interaction. You move, during sleep, beyond time and space.

The drive to regain full consciousness or full awareness heightens in many individuals who experience Reiki. In Second Degree Reiki classes you are taught how to do a Second Degree Reiki treatment on others and on yourself. Most students of Reiki further explore its usefulness. They do treatments regularly after learning the symbols and having the energy transmissions. Thus, the richness of Reiki reveals itself many times over.

The Self communicates with/to you in symbolic form because symbols carry a richness that transcends time, space, and words.

The symbols of dreams often depict awareness that emerges from deep layers of your being. The educated observer recognizes that they occur cross-culturally as well as through the ages historically. Thus, a dream may carry an image that, when expanded, reveals an image that another dreamer, in another time and place also had. These images come out of the depths of your psyche; they have energy that often carries a great deal of power. Jung called such images archetypes and contrasted them to images that relate only to your personal emotional life.

WHAT REIKI CAN DO FOR YOU IN THE FOUR WORLDS

In order for you to feel whole, you must function in a harmonious way. When any part of you moves out of sync or out of alignment, you are likely to feel the shift and must adapt or compensate in some manner to accommodate it. I have documented what esoteric literature generally describes as your body functioning in four interrelated worlds, often described as four interrelated bodies that work together as an integrated unified whole. These bodies are:

Your Physical Body

This body corresponds to your experienced physical body. Your physical body exists and interacts with the objective physical world of life and/or reality. In addition, your cells, your physiology, your brain, and your movements all function on this physical level, often without conscious intervention on your part. Think about the automatic way your body digests food, functions when you sleep, or "knows what to do" when you walk or move.

Your Spiritual Body

This body refers to your energy experience of connectedness between cosmic forces of the universe and how you manifest this energy in the physical world. Through this spiritual (or etheric) world, all life connects. A full experience of your spiritual body allows you to experience the interconnectedness of all life and its unity. The kind of kinship you feel with those you love, the unity of human compassion that draws and drives you forward toward something greater than yourself constitutes the spiritual body. It is often experienced as an inner Knowing. I call it Knowing with a "K".

Your Emotional Body

This body carries your feelings that convey positive or negative charges of energy. Your issues deriving from personal experiences may become fixed in your emotional (or astral) body. Distress may arise because emotional reactions are often based in desires rather than in factual analysis of situations. When you are not congruently aligned with your higher Self or life purpose, you are likely to feel disharmony and discomfort. When you feel dissonance and ill at ease, use the power of your self-talk to reframe your thinking in ways that shift your feelings so they better align with your values and thus, they empower you.

Your Mental Body

This body carries thought patterns, interconnections, and associations based on analysis and understanding of the outer world. The component elements of consciousness get carried and integrated into the physical world through your mind. This body operates in the reality of your life interactions, making you vulnerable to environmental circumstances and how they affect your thinking. Taking dominion over this energy body is essential to balance because through it you have the power within your own mind to change thought patterns and belief systems that influence interactions in your life.

Summary: The Four Energy Bodies

These four energy bodies function together as a whole. Awareness of Self as a whole and consciousness of various energy bodies can be helpful in pinpointing areas of particular strength or areas within you that lack clarity. When the four energy bodies work as an integrated whole, you feel life energy flowing smoothly—you feel a sense of well-being, i.e., happiness and health. Any disturbance in a particular "body" creates a sense of disturbance through your whole being. Go to: https://www.nobleenergywellness.com/summary-manifest-your-dreams-2023-08-03/ for more information on how these bodies function in you and to see how all systems of esoteric knowledge integrate into a unified system.

WHAT EACH DEGREE OF REIKI DOES

While First Degree Reiki is a hands-on treatment, it opens the door for you to perceive subtle energy levels that flow through, around, and between you and others. With Second Degree Reiki, you learn symbols that activate your capacity to do energy transmissions at a distance and across time.

All Reiki levels give you the opportunity to harmonize your energetic bodies in an integrated way. As you do Reiki treatments, you receive the energy via your Crown Chakra, through your body, and out your hands. Reiki energies touch all levels simultaneously. Thus, it allows you to expand awareness of how you function. Your expanded awareness will become clearer to you as you do more treatments, and it may be used to accomplish an understanding of how you organize resources in your Self to manifest in the world.

CHAKRAS

Chakras have been described as energy centers in the body. In the Hindu Chakra System, seven major chakras have been described: the base/root chakra, the sexual/sensational chakra, the solar plexus chakra, the heart chakra, the throat chakra, the third eye chakra, and the crown chakra (illustration below). Each chakra centers in a different part of your body and relates to different aspects of your evolving consciousness.

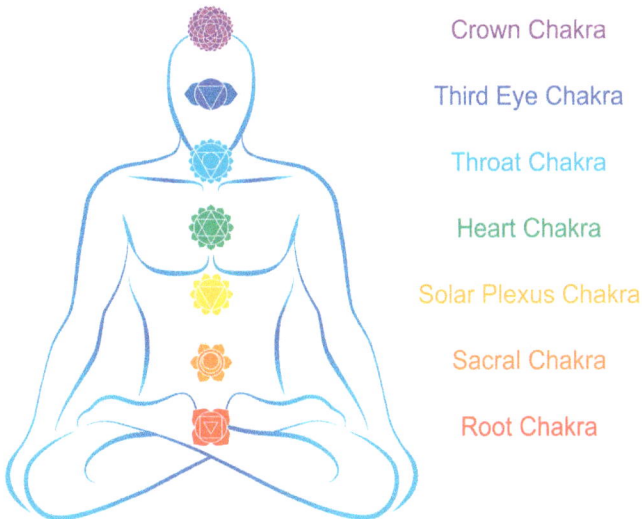

Crown Chakra

Third Eye Chakra

Throat Chakra

Heart Chakra

Solar Plexus Chakra

Sacral Chakra

Root Chakra

The Hindu Chakra System

KABALISTIC TREE OF LIFE

In the Kabalistic Tree of Life, energy centers are called Sephiroth. In the Tree of Life (illustration below), there are ten designated energy centers that connect through thirty-two paths of intelligence describing the process of evolving consciousness. As each task or path is completed in each of the four energy bodies, or worlds, as they are called in the Tree of Life, new awareness and discernment of subtleties of functioning become active.

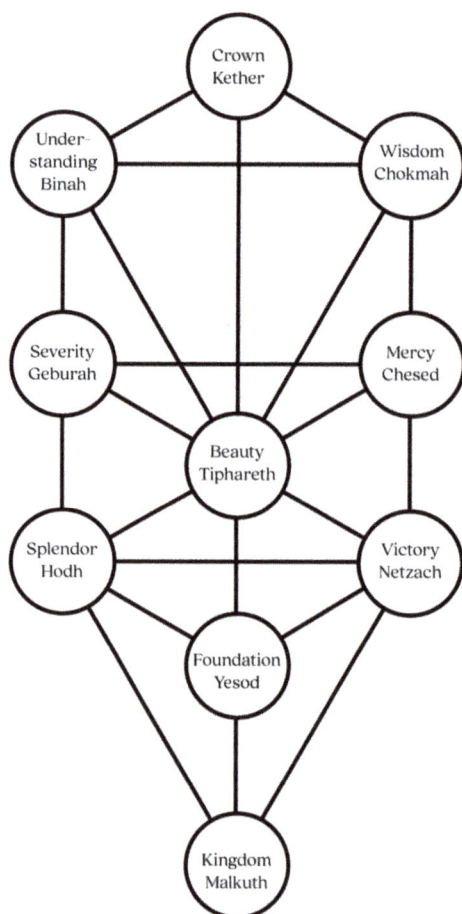

The Tree of Life

As you explore your chakras and/or Sephiroth (paths of intelligence) using Reiki you will be amazed, I am sure, to learn that your awareness and feelings mirror those of sages through the ages. You will tap into archetypal (collective group) levels of awareness in a very direct way. The experience of these dimensions will open you in unexpected ways.

PSYCHOLOGICAL TYPES

Another structural dimension of your personality may be tapped by delving into what C.G. Jung described as your psychological type. Your "psychological type" describes the main way you process and organize information about the world and about your Self. Jung described four functions that encompass ways of perceiving or judging information about the world. He also described two primary attitudinal modes of organizing these functions.

The four functions and their organization in your personality determine your psychological type. Thus, you may be either predominantly an extrovert or predominantly an introvert. An extrovert directs energy outward from the Self toward the objective world. Relationships in the world show in your expression of your Self. As an introvert you take energy inward toward your subjective world; your relationship with your inner world determines self-experience. Within the framework of these two primary attitude modes of organizing energy, you have a dominant function type. The functions are: intuition, sensation, thinking, and feeling.

Expansion of these types and an actual energy description of how you function may be learned from my work. I developed and scientifically documented my work through Noble Energy Wellness, using multidimensional tools that describe Five Ways of Being (Types) and their functioning (https://www.nobleenergywellness. com/the-5-types/). You can learn a great deal about your communication patterns as well as about the perceptive or judging filters you impose upon the world and upon others through studying this information. In addition, when you treat your "functional typology" you begin a process that develops functions that you generally put in a secondary position within your Self. Through my work in Noble Sciences, I statistically documented five types on over 45,000 cases.

The five types are: Manifestor, Generator, Manifesting Generator, the Projector, and Reflector. These types correspond to Jungian types with the Manifesting Generator serving as an Integrative Type. The Manifesting Generator uses more than one strategy in functioning. The Manifestor is the Thinking Type, the Generator is the Feeling Type, the Projector is the Sensation Type, and the Reflector is the Intuitive Type.

You are about 99% likely to become a Manifesting Generator i.e., someone who can make things happen when unconscious and conscious intention align and come to fruition in the world of form, when you live in your integrated auric energy field. (Research done by Eleanor Haspel-Portner, Ph.D. through Noble Sciences, LLC.) Thus, Noble Sciences considers more than just your conscious and unconscious worlds that define waking consciousness.

In addition, Noble Energy Maps provide you with an actual body energy map from which you can see your mechanical (genetic) structure. By working with Reiki on your actual body energy map you can bring about great awareness and change using any degree of Reiki energy to bypass the issues of your personality.

By doing the treatments on your attitude and on how you function, you may learn a great deal about how these aspects work in you. To get a copy of your free Energy Map log in to http://www.nobleenergywellness.com/energy-map/ with your birth date, time, and place of birth and receive your personalized map.

Reiki, at any level of initiation, begins a deep process of self-exploration as well as activating lifelong healing energy. The white light healing energy activated in your hands turns on and flows whenever you touch any living being. Once this process is activated by a certified Usui Reiki Master/Teacher, you have the energy for life, and the more consciously you use it, the more benefit you will reap from it. As with any self-growth or healing modality, setting your intention on using the energy for the highest good, and never imposing will or specifics that may influence the higher purpose at hand, is essential to optimal healing.

REIKI FACTS SUMMARIZED

What Reiki Is

Reiki, a natural pure white light healing energy, is channeled through an individual who has been personally initiated into Reiki. The Reiki initiation is a hands-on process that involves a series of four "attunements." The Reiki Master/Teacher uses a specific formula for each Reiki attunement and each attunement is done exactly as originally taught by Dr. Usui. The Reiki Initiation activates and sets the Reiki energy path in motion within the initiated individual.

The Reiki energy path runs through an individual's crown chakra through their Satsuma, the central energy channel along the spinal column activating the chakra system and centering in the heart chakra. From the heart center, the energy flows through the hands.

Whenever a Reiki initiated individual touches anything alive, Reiki energy automatically flows through the individual's hands without additional effort or expenditure of energy.

Because of the purity of the energy, when doing a treatment no negative energy can be picked up by the healer and taken into their body so no protection is necessary.

What Reiki Does

One of the aspects of Reiki that sets it apart from many other healing modalities is the fact that in Reiki, the energy that flows is independent of the clarity or of the healing ability of the person doing the healing work. Because Reiki is a pure white light energy, the healer is only a conduit for positive white light energy; no negative energy can be transferred through the healer.

In other healing modalities, differences often exist in the intensity and in the energy level of the individual doing the healing work. In Reiki, the power of the energy transmission varies based only on the level of Reiki to which the healer has been attuned or initiated. The Reiki healer needs no protection from negative forces or energies and does not need to center and/or to focus meditatively when engaging in healing work in order to keep it pure. Reiki remains a pure energy regardless of the consciousness, physical, emotional, or mental state of the healer. This purity of Reiki and its transmission sets it apart from other healing modalities.

What Makes Reiki Special

Reiki brings about the alignment of the physical and emotional energies in individuals through the transmission of pure white light energy that flows through the Reiki practitioner's hands as soon as they touch a living being. The energy releases physical and emotional energies and, thus, promotes harmony and balance. Individuals who study Reiki always have an empowering tool in their hands that they can use to shift their consciousness and grow toward wholeness and health.

Because Reiki increases one's sense of power by maintaining a connection with the Universal Life Force at all times, it is a cost-effective way to enhance the immune system and attain optimal health. Because the power of Reiki is in the hands, no tools or shifts of consciousness are required to turn the energy flow on. Thus, even in times of emergencies, Reiki is available to those initiated in the energy. Reiki is a white light energy and requires no special belief system and is not a religion. Anyone can be initiated into Reiki. Often in my practice of Reiki, I have given newborns the gift of Reiki.

REIKI LEVELS AND INITIATION

The Reiki Initiation Process

Once you are initiated into Reiki, you have the energy flowing through your hands for the rest of your life. Thus, an initiation into any degree of Reiki is a serious undertaking and should be treated as such. Reiki must be activated in an initiation by a Reiki Master/ Teacher to a Reiki Student. It is done individually, ideally in person, but it can be done at distance. Reiki can only be transferred/

learned in this way. The Reiki initiation process is a very exact and specific formula.

Part of the process of becoming a Reiki Master/Teacher is understanding the specifics of the initiation process and their commitment to keep the initiation constant and unmodified. The Reiki Master/Teacher uses the exact form as passed down by Dr. Usui, the founder of Reiki, and by Mrs. Takata who brought Reiki to the West. As in any true initiation process, the Reiki Master/Teacher is only important for his/her professional adherence to the integrity of the system. The individual personality of the Reiki Master/Teacher is irrelevant in the process.

Each level of Reiki power is complete in itself so that no other attunement or process is required once the process of initiation is completed at a given Reiki level of power. The energy path during an initiation is set for life; it remains active whenever the individual with Reiki touches a living being including plants and animals. The energy always remains active in an individual once that individual is initiated. A true Reiki Master/Teacher does not upsell you to other levels of initiation.

There are Three Levels of Reiki Initiations

First Degree Reiki activates healing energy that flows when any living being is physically touched.

Second Degree Reiki heightens the power of First Degree Reiki energy tenfold. Second Degree Reiki activates healing energy, so it flows when certain symbols are activated by the Reiki practitioner. The Reiki Symbols activate healing at-a-distance, i.e., the person receiving the Reiki treatment need not be physically present to receive it. The energy accesses the mental, emotional, spiritual, and physical aspects of an individual and heals on all those levels of being.

Third Degree Reiki heightens the power of Second Degree Reiki energy tenfold. Third Degree Reiki activates healing energy that sets the Reiki path in motion in another individual and operates on a deep level of co-creation. Third Degree Reiki allows the Reiki Master/Teacher to initiate others into Reiki. The process of becoming a Reiki Master/Teacher is a lifelong commitment and requires study of healing principles, working with the Reiki energy, apprenticing with a Reiki Master/Teacher to learn exactly how to do the attunements and understand the nuances of the experiences that teachers have when initiating their students into Reiki energy. The process of a Reiki initiation is detailed, and each initiation has a unique flow of energy interaction with the initiate. This process is important to understand when studying Third Degree Reiki.

THE REIKI PRINCIPLES

These are principles that every Reiki initiate lives by. When initiated into Reiki at any degree, the student is asked to memorize these Reiki principles and to repeat them as affirmations daily.

1. Just for today, I count my many blessings and show gratitude.
2. Just for today, I will not worry.
3. Just for today, I shall not anger.
4. Just for today, I will earn my livelihood honestly.
5. Just for today, I will be kind to all life and all creation.

♦ ♦ ♦

THE REIKI TREATMENT AND HAND POSITIONS

DOING A FIRST-DEGREE REIKI TREATMENT

Once you have gone through your Reiki Attunement and have active Reiki energy in your hands when you touch any living being, you are ready to do Reiki treatments on yourself and on other people, plants, and animals.

In order to do a Reiki treatment, you do not need any preparation and your state of mind is not relevant to the treatment. The pure white light energy of Reiki will flow from your hands upon touching a living being.

To prepare for a treatment, make sure you and whomever you are treating is in a comfortable setting and can remain undisturbed. The treatment takes about an hour. Before starting, wash your hands and make sure you are well-hydrated.

In a Reiki Treatment, there are four Head positions, five Front Positions, and five Back Position. In addition, there are a few additional hands-on positions specific to a man or a woman, highlighting areas where additional healing frequency energy is welcomed.

The positions in this manual are laid out for easy reference and include notes from my initial First Degree Reiki Class with Mrs. Takata present in June, 1977. At the time of the class, I did not know anything about Reiki, but I knew that having Mrs. Takata at the class was important. Thus, during the class I took copious notes and learned some nuances that Mrs. Takata shared from her years of treating people using Reiki.

I have incorporated all my notes so they are easy to read and keep for quick reference, covering all the Reiki positions as well as some additional positions that are helpful to know and use.

When doing a treatment, the fingers are always together, and the hands are next to each other as in the diagrams illustrating each Reiki position. With First Degree Reiki, it is necessary to stay on each position for 5 minutes. At the end of the 5 minutes, move to the next position. Always treat using all the positions, and if there is an issue, e.g., knee pain, go to the that specific area after you finish all the other positions. The reason for this is that you want to treat the whole person and the source of the issue which may not have originated in the painful area.

It is also important to note that it is not necessary to physically touch the person you are working on. You can hold your hand slightly above the body and the energy will penetrate as though your hand is on the body. People are often aware of the energy flow.

You do not have to focus or concentrate during a treatment. Thus, you can do treatments on yourself when you are watching television, stopping at traffic lights, or even sitting in a classroom listening to a lecture. The main point is to use your Reiki healing hands as much and as often as you can to reap the most benefit.

Reiki Head Positions

The First Head Position has the following benefits in each of Field of Awareness

Rejuvenates your body through the pituitary gland, the master gland that balances hormones. Use this position when you want to clear your head and refocus in a relaxed way. This position is very important for diabetics.

MENTAL WORLD

Enhances clarity
Focuses thoughts
Focuses feelings
Relaxes your mind
Focuses concentration
Maximizes centering

SPIRITUAL WORLD

Activates the Sixth Chakra (The Third Eye Center).

Allows knowing and vision to expand
into another dimension

Helps in meditation to open the Crown Center

First Head Position

**Position Hands Together,
Thumbs Toward Ears**

Dark Blue Represents the Ajna Chakra

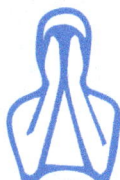

EMOTIONAL WORLD

Calms your mind
Turns your focus inward
Relaxes your mind and body
Shuts out external stimuli
Reduces overall stress

PHYSICAL WORLD

Balances the hypothalamus and pituitary glands

Helps:
Eyes, Sinus, Nose, and Allergy problems

Improves and helps heal:
Teeth, Upper Jaw, Ear Problems, Vertigo

Reiki Head Positions

The Second Head Position has the following benefits in each of Field of Awareness

Rejuvenates your body through balancing the hemispheres of the brain, resulting in clarity and focus of thoughts and relief from anxiety and stress. When your brain hemispheres are balanced, your calm, clear thinking is enhanced. Use this position when you have difficulty focusing and need clarity of mind.

MENTAL WORLD

Helps:

Balance your brain hemispheres
Enhance memory
Mental clarity

Clear depression
Increase alertness
Heighten creativity
Integrate thought

SPIRITUAL WORLD

Activates:
The Crown Chakra
Higher awareness
Expanded consciousness

Enhances:
Clarity of mind
Awareness
Psychic openness

Second Head Position

**Palms at Temples,
Fingers Together at Crown**

Purple Represents the Crown Chakra

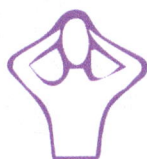

EMOTIONAL WORLD

Helps:

Relieve stress and worry
Calm anxiety
Decrease depression
Enhance dream recall

Centering
Focus your mind
Balance the hemispheres
of your brain

PHYSICAL WORLD

Works on:
Pituitary and pineal glands (from lateral angle)

Helps:

Headaches
Dizziness
Shock

Motion sickness
Pain
TMJ

Facilitates the release of endorphins.

Reiki Head Positions

The Third Head Position has the following benefits in each of Field of Awareness

Rejuvenates and balances your body through the hypothalamus, the center of the brain that regulates the autonomous nervous system. This position helps with overall well-being and is especially helpful in falling asleep and in remembering dreams. It activates the cranial and vagus nerves.

MENTAL WORLD

Helps:
Balance your autonomic nervous system
Build your sense of well-being
Relaxed comfort
Reduce pain
Facilitate dream recall

SPIRITUAL WORLD

Balances mental well-being
Regulates the release of hypothalamic hormones

Enhances:
Clear expression of thoughts
Clear expression of ideas

Increases productivity

Expands multidimensional consciousness

Third Head Position

Fingers Together at Back of Head, Palms at Base of Head

Dark Blue Represents the Ajna Chakra

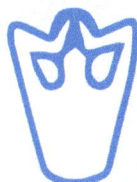

EMOTIONAL WORLD

Activates the back of your head to balance your
third eye center for increased awareness

Enhances:
Perceptual awareness and receptivity of higher energies
Processing of higher energy frequencies
with increased ease and comfort

PHYSICAL WORLD

Works on hypothalamus:
Controls autonomic processes such as
blood presure, heartbeat, breathing

Helps:
Weight loss
Improve balance and coordination
Facilitate sleep induction
Relieve headaches

Reiki Head Positions

The Fourth Head Position has the following benefits in each of Field of Awareness

Rejuvenates your body through your thyroid and parathyroid glands, the master glands for balancing your metabolism and blood pressure. Since your Throat is the Power center for manifestation in the world, balancing this center enhances self-expression and self-esteem. Higher consciousness is enhanced in this position. If you have difficulty expressing yourself, energizing your throat may breakdown your fears and resistance to speaking. This position is important for lymphatic drainage.

MENTAL WORLD

Helps:
Balance your throat
Bring clarity of expression

Stabilizes:
The connection of your words with thoughts

Allows:
Your clarity to manifest

SPIRITUAL WORLD

Builds up:
Throat as a power for your center of communication
and creative expression
Higher energies that gain expression through your throat,
enhancing their manifestation

Fourth Head Position

Hands Around Throat

Light Blue Represents the
Throat Chakra

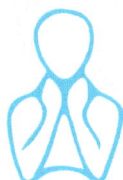

EMOTIONAL WORLD

Balances:
Metabolism
Circulation

Helps:

Control anger
Increase self-esteem

Enhance empowered feelings
Enhance self-confidence

Facilitates:
Release of pent-up emotions

PHYSICAL WORLD

Helps:

Thyroid functioning
Parathyroid functioning
Balance metabolism
Regulate blood pressure

Throat issues
Tonsil, adenoid problems
Allergies
Bronchial problems

Activates:
Thymus gland and lymphatic system drainage

Reiki Front Positions

**The First Front Position has the following benefits
in each of Field of Awareness**

Because this position works on your heart, lungs, and thymus gland, it opens you to your soul connection with the Divine. The more you experience this connection, the easier it becomes to recognize it in others. Reiki energy flows through the Heart Center in a frequency of Divine love and light. Balancing through a Reiki treatment opens you to experience the healing love of the Divine.

MENTAL WORLD

Helps:
Harmonious attitudes
Center thoughts and images
Brings you an integrative sense of clarity

SPIRITUAL WORLD

Opens your Heart Chakra to love
that transcends the personal level of your being

Connects you with the soul level of others
and with their higher selves

First Front Position

**Hands at Level of Heart,
Fingertips Touching**

Green Represents the Heart Chakra

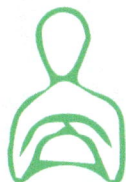

EMOTIONAL WORLD

Works on:
Heart center

Builds:
Trust
Courage
Positive self-esteem

Balances:
Anger
Negative feelings

Promotes:
Good feelings
Loving feelings

Reduces sadness

PHYSICAL WORLD

Works on:
Heart and lungs
Circulation
Thymus gland, positively affecting the immune system

Relieves:
Asthma
Chest wall pressure and pain

The Second Front Position has the following benefits in each of Field of Awareness

Realigns and balances your Solar Plexus Chakra including major organs of digestion and detoxification. When balanced, you are likely to experience more clarity and freedom from daily stressors. You are likely to experience more even emotional responses and less reactivity. When you have digestive issues, this position may be helpful.

MENTAL WORLD

Releases:
Power motive
Anger

Helps:
Mental clarity through centering
Cleansing your body of cloudy thoughts
related to bodily functions
Foster kindness

SPIRITUAL WORLD

Opens you to their your power
without the need for control

Respects your individual control or free choice

Facilitates your acceptance of the
ebb and flow of life energies

Second Front Position

**Hand Under Breast,
Fingertips Touching**

Yellow Represents the Solar Plexus Chakra

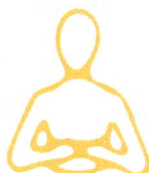

EMOTIONAL WORLD

Eases:

Fears   Negativity

Releases:
Stress generated by your body functions
Need to be in control of things

Promotes relaxation

PHYSICAL WORLD

Covers major organs:

Liver   Pancreas
Spleen   Gall bladder
Stomach

Helps:
Digestion
Detoxification and processes of major body functions
Relieve digestive discomfort

Reiki Front Positions

The Third Front Position has the following benefits in each of Field of Awareness

Balances the Lower part of your Solar Plexus Chakra that includes your liver and the stomach. Digestive issues relax and release through treatments on this area. As your body releases tension in this area of your body, your mental fogginess and tiredness diminish.

MENTAL WORLD

Helps:
Clear your body of fogginess that
interferes with mental clarity

Clears:
Depression
Confusion

SPIRITUAL WORLD

Your Solar Plexus Chakra helps:
Release your need for control or for acceptance
Keep your focus on the present moment
Release your past associations that hinder conscious living

Third Front Position

Hands Just Above the Waist
Fingers Touching

Yellow Represents the Solar Plexus Chakra

EMOTIONAL WORLD

Builds:
Self-confidence
Relaxation

Reduces Stress:
Releases your need for control or for acceptance
Facilitates your acceptance of self and others
Releases past associations that interfere with the present

PHYSICAL WORLD

Covers:
Lower part of your liver
Small and large intestines
Lower stomach

Relaxes and aids your digestion

Reduces pain from indigestion

Reiki Front Positions

The Fourth Front Position has the following benefits in each of Field of Awareness

Focused energy in your pelvis balances your sexual organs as well as your large and small intestines. When in equilibrium, your sense of adaptability and flexibility allow you to be creative and related to others. Your energy field becomes more powerful in attracting what you need. Sexual energy flows from this chakra. Use this position to help with menstrual cramps.

MENTAL WORLD

Increases:
Your Flexibility of thinking
Your adaptability

Releases:
Fear
Rigidity

SPIRITUAL WORLD

Focuses energy on:
Pelvic, Sexual Chakra

Opens you to the connections and relatedness of energy vibrations between living things
Magnetizes your energy field

Fourth Front Position

Hands Below The Waist
Fingers Touching

Orange Represents the Sex Chakra

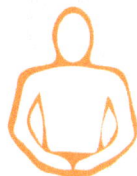

EMOTIONAL WORLD

Frees your sexual energy from conditioned patterns
Alleviates your fears and anxiety
Builds your confidence

PHYSICAL WORLD

Covers:
Pelvis
Ovaries and uterus
Prostate
Bladder
Large and small intestines

Helps:
Release toxins
Migraines associated with digestive imbalances
Constipation and diarrhea
Abdominal pain

Reiki Front Positions

The Fifth Front Position has the following benefits in each of Field of Awareness

The Root Chakra is the foundation from which you operate, it relates to your values and your strength, and it is the basis of your self-esteem and confidence. Circulation is enhanced in this position and thus, as Reiki energy moves through you, it clears any blockages and frees you up to take a stand that aligns with your core being.

MENTAL WORLD

Clarifies your assumptions that form the foundation of your thinking

Rids you of negative debris

SPIRITUAL WORLD

The Root Chakra anchors and supports your physical well-being

Important in clearing your body so your foundation is firm

Fifth Front Position

Hands Over Groin
V-Shaped Fingers Touching
Red Represents the Root Chakra

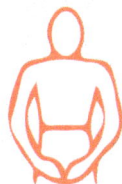

EMOTIONAL WORLD

Helps:
Build your confidence
Self-esteem

Clarifies values which are important to you
and that form the basis of your feelings

PHYSICAL WORLD

Covers:
Root position over groin

Builds:
Physical strength by generating energy through
the base of your trunk

Works on:
Genitals
Groin area
Circulation to your legs (leg lymphatics)

Reiki Back Positions

The First Back Position has the following benefits in each of Field of Awareness

Relaxation and release from your neck and throat allow energy to move more freely through your body reducing inflammation and pain and connecting mind and body in ways that enhance your overall well-being and communication. Sitting with your hand on your neck in this position can be very freeing and relaxing. Use it often.

MENTAL WORLD

Works on:
Relaxation
Centering
Clarity of expression
Collects your thoughts for mental stability

SPIRITUAL WORLD

Balances:
Throat Chakra
The nervous system

Overall:
Connects your mind and body
Sense of your integration of being
All communication is enhanced

First Back Position

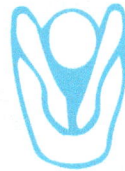

EMOTIONAL WORLD

Facilitates:
Tension release
Stress reduction
Control of anger
Increase in your self esteem

Release of pent up emotion resulting in:
Positive feelings
Self-confidence
Freedom of your mind to deal with feelings

PHYSICAL WORLD

Relaxes:
Neck and trapezius
Upper lungs
Upper spinal cord (C7-T4)

Reduces pain and inflammation
from tight muscles and joints

Reiki Back Positions

The Second Back Position has the following benefits in each of Field of Awareness

Relaxed breathing from the enhanced energy of Reiki allows your heart to open and your circulatory system to flow. When you feel that your thoughts can flow freely, you are likely to feel empowered and clear. Note: This is a difficult position to do on yourself. To make it easier use one hand at a time. Because it activates the lungs it is an important position to work at.

MENTAL WORLD

Clears your mind by freeing your body of impurities in your circulatory system

Helps you feel like thoughts can travel through the air

SPIRITUAL WORLD

Activates:
Your Heart Chakra

Lets you open to the energy around and to respond with a clear sense of yourself

Second Back Position

Hand on Lower Shoulder
Next to Spine

Green Represents The Heart Chakra

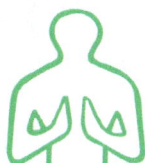

EMOTIONAL WORLD

Relaxes tension almost immediately.

Lets you catch your breath
so you can handle whatever is before you

Helps:
Center and calm your emotions
Build courage

PHYSICAL WORLD

Helps:
Lungs, heart, circulation
Energy in your body
Breathing

Your left shoulder relaxes:
Your body
Your nervous system

Your right shoulder helps:
Gall bladder
Enhances sleep
Heart and lung conditions

Reiki Back Positions

The Third Back Position has the following benefits in each of Field of Awareness

Energy flows into your kidney and adrenal glands, helping manage stress and relieving any confusion, fears, and toxicity in your body. This position is easy to do on yourself when you are waiting in lines. Trust is enhanced in this position as is the impulse toward action. By working on this position extra, you build more adrenal resilience.

MENTAL WORLD

Helps clear your mind by relieving it of:
Confusion
Extraneous thoughts, fears, angst

Enhances:
Clarity
Logic

SPIRITUAL WORLD

Builds a sense of ability to:
Take action
Accomplish things

Helps you feel:
Trusting and confident
In touch with higher energies
In touch with your purposes

Third Back Position

**Small of Back
Fingers Touching**

Yellow Represents the Solar Plexus Chakra

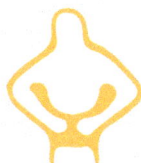

EMOTIONAL WORLD

Relieves stress
Releases fear

Helps you feel:
Secure
Trusting

Balances your emotions

PHYSICAL WORLD

Helps:
Kidneys and adrenal glands   Immune system
Pancreas and liver   Shock and whiplash

Gives you increased stamina

Very important position for:
Clearing your body of toxins
Handling stress

Reiki Back Positions

The Fourth Back Position has the following benefits in each of Field of Awareness

Security and trust gain energy from activating this chakra and its meridians. Balancing your nervous system enhances your immune system and builds clarity and life force energy. This position is near the "Gate of Life" a key area in the back where the energy moves up your body. Energy in this area of the back is important for opening your consciousness.

MENTAL WORLD

Helps clear your mind by relieving it of:
Confusion
Extraneous thoughts

Enhances:
Clarity
Logic

SPIRITUAL WORLD

Works on:
Solar Plexus Chakra
Generating primal energy

Used As:
Life force energy
Energy that forms as the foundation of all action

Fourth Back Position

Base of spine forming V

Orange Represents the Sex Chakra

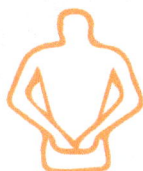

EMOTIONAL WORLD

Opens you to your own base of energy

Generates:
Security
Trust and integrity

From this point emerges greater energy

PHYSICAL WORLD

Base of your spine, coccyx

Helps your nervous system:
Balance energy
Generate chi energy

Energizes and builds:
Sexual function
Stamina

Reiki Back Positions

The Fifth Back Position has the following benefits in each of Field of Awareness

Comfort and security become more stable, and you are energized to keep grounded when Reiki activates the Root Chakra. Security comes from your inner confidence that you are balanced and calm. Using this position strengthens your ability to stand your ground.

MENTAL WORLD

Calms your mind
Calm and soothing energy

Gives:
Confidence
Ease to thinking

SPIRITUAL WORLD

Works:
Through your Root Chakra

Enhances:
Your grounding process
Security of being

Balances your physical body

Fifth Back Position

On Buttocks

Red Represents the Root Chakra

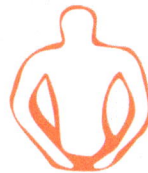

EMOTIONAL WORLD

Low key enhancement of:
Security
Confidence

Not an action oriented position

PHYSICAL WORLD

Works on:
The buttocks

Promotes:
Sense of comfort   Sense of security

Helps:
Warm your body   Relaxation and sleep

Good for:
Stroke   Bedridden
Sciatica

♦ ♦ ♦

CULTIVATING YOUR PRACTICE OF REIKI

When Reiki enters your life, it changes you in amazing ways. Learning Reiki primarily involves receiving an energy transmission known as an attunement, thus, you may be somewhat nonchalant about what has just happened to you at a deep level of your consciousness. A Reiki attunement activates an already flowing channel in your energy body. As time passes and you use your Reiki, consciously or unconsciously, your powerful flow of energy or chi increases, and with it so does the awareness of your healing capacity.

You live in an energy body in a third dimensional world. The third dimensional world surrounds you as a concrete existence, and it is the world in which you relate to others in daily life without considering the multifaceted components of every interaction.

As you open to the energy frequencies of healing, the fourth, fifth, and dimensions beyond will open to you, because your consciousness will be open to perceive these worlds and energies.

A First Degree Reiki treatment takes an hour because you have 14 hand positions, and each requires 5 minutes for a full treatment. Often, a First Degree Reiki initiate does a self-treatment in the course of a 24-hour day. Over time, the accumulated benefits become apparent, and your perception of subtle energies around people you encounter or come close to begins to surface into your ordinary awareness.

Everyone experiences Reiki in their unique way.

Pay attention to your senses: hearing, seeing, touching, tasting, smelling.

- What differences do you notice in any of these senses since studying Reiki?

- When you do a Reiki Treatment on yourself, what do you notice?

- When you do a Reiki Treatment on someone else, what do you notice?

  » Is there any sensation in your hands?

  » Do you sense any differences in the areas you put your hands on?

  » What difference do you notice in yourself from before, during, and after the treatment?

Recording the answers to questions such as these in a journal with your observations helps document your experiences and also may reveal more growth and awareness in you than you acknowledge in your daily life. Take this opportunity to grow and expand your consciousness.

Because the power of each level of Reiki increases ten times, I highly recommend that you invest in becoming a Second Degree Reiki practitioner. The cost is set by the Reiki Alliance and is followed by all Reiki Practitioners. If you wish to proceed with your study of either First or Second Degree Reiki, please use the Reiki

Alliance Directory to find a qualified and vetted Reiki Master/ Teacher to do the initiations or attunements.

If you wish to have me or Marvin initiate you, we are happy to do so in person or via a zoom call where we do the actual attunement at a distance. We can record the call so you can review and share your experience later.

♦ ♦ ♦

THE REIKI STORY

R eiki has been passed down as an oral tradition. What I know of the story is based on what I heard from Mrs. Takata, the recounting of the story by Virginia Samdahl, and information from the Reiki Alliance. I am including the combined details, despite the repetition because they are of historic significance.

THE HISTORY OF REIKI AND ITS LINEAGE

Around the turn of the century a man named Dr. Mikao Usui, was president and minster of a Christian school in Kyoto, Japan. One morning after the daily message, some of Dr. Usui's graduating seniors came forward and said to him:

"Do you accept the contents of the Bible literally?" Dr. Usui said he did.

His students then asked him if he believed what the Bible said about Jesus healing the sick and walking on water and they asked if he had ever seen these miracles happen. Dr. Usui was unable to personally validate healings and other "miracles." And his students were asking for evidence before they could fully commit to believe the bible and to go out into the world on healing missions.

Dr. Usui committed to find the key to healing miracles. He traveled to the University of Chicago where he received a doctorate in scripture hoping to find the secret to Jesus' healing the sick. He was disappointed that he did not find what he wanted to know.

He returned to Japan and continued to seek his answers. He studied Sanskrit, hoping the language would allow him to find his answer, but did not find the clues he sought. After seven years, he came to the last monastery, back in Kyoto. When he asked to see the bishop of that monastery, a tiny man about 72 years old with a little round baby face came forth.

Dr. Usui asked if he knew how to heal the body. "Does the Zen know how to heal the body?"

The bishop responded, "No longer."

Usui said, "No longer? You mean at one time this temple knew how to heal the body!"

And he said, "Oh yes. But we discovered that when we healed the body, the man was sick of spirit. He was not whole. So, we spent so much time healing the spirit, we've forgotten how to heal the body. And we find that when we heal the spirit and don't heal the body, the man's not whole. But now we don't know how to heal the body anymore."

Mount Kurama-yama is a large holy mountain north of Kyoto. Usui swung around and faced Mount Kurama-yama, and threw up his hands and said, "This is the end! This is the last place I had to search. All these years, and there's no place else to go! I am through. I am finished."

And the little monk said, "Usui Sensei, forgive me for speaking. But I must tell you the Zen never say, "This is the end." We always say, "This is the beginning. And we believe that when one door closes another one opens. And I believe that if you are truly dedicated, and if you do not give up in your quest, you will again learn how to heal the body. Because if it was once known, it can be known again."

And Dr. Usui questioned, "You truly believe this?"

He replied, "I do, or I would not say this to you."

Dr. Usui said, "You're the only one who has ever given me any hope. May I study with you?"

"Of course, All are welcomed by the Zen."

Dr. Usui moved into that monastery and had a small room there. For three years, from early in the morning at first light until it was so dark you could read no longer, he read the sutras in Japanese.

He remembered what the little monk had told him and resolved "If I don't find it, I'm not going deep enough. And I'm determined I am going to find the answer! All the great scholars' study in Chinese. I will learn Chinese!" And he did. He took his doctorate in Chinese until he could read and understand to perfection. Again, for three years, from the first light until dark he read the sutras in Chinese – and found nothing. And he thought, "I will not give up! I am not going deep enough. Buddhism came to us from India, so I will learn Sanskrit."

And he did. He learned Sanskrit until he could read and understand it to perfection. Then he started to read the sutras in original Sanskrit. And in that language, he found the key. He found the key to healing the body.

Of course, he was ecstatic! He rushed to the new bishop, (since the little old bishop of years before had passed over). But the new bishop was as interested in what Dr. Usui was doing as the old bishop. So Usui said to him. "Look!!! I have found the keys. I have found how to do this thing. They talk about the power, but how am I going to gain the power?"

The bishop suggested, "I think first we should meditate and pray," and Usui agreed.

So, they both went to their rooms after dinner that night, and each in his own way meditated and prayed on how Usui was to find the power. They came together after breakfast the next morning. And it was decided that Usui should go out to the Mount Kurama-yama to a specific level facing east, and for 21 days and nights he should fast and meditate. They were hopeful that something would be shown to him.

Dr. Usui got himself ready, and as he was leaving the compound that morning, there was a little eight-year-old boy from the monastery at the gate. Usui looked down at that little fellow and said, "Son, I'm going out to Mount Kurama-yama and I'm going to fast and meditate for 21 days and nights. And I should be back here at twilight on the twenty-first day. But if I'm not, then you come out the morning of the twenty-second day and get my bones—because I'm dead."

And the little boy said, "Yes sir, Usui Sensei! I will do that."

And Dr. Usui went the seventeen and a half miles to his appointed place on Mount Kurama-yama. When he arrived there, he realized he had no watch and no calendar. So, he gathered up 21 small stones and piled them up in front of him. And each morning as he began his meditation, he'd pick up a stone and throw it away. And that's how he kept his calendar.

He later told one of his students, Dr. Chujiro Hayashi, whom he later appointed head of the Masters as his successor, "You know, you have heard it said it is so dark before the dawn? It is true.

It's so dark you cannot see your hand in front of your face. That is true. Because on the twenty-first day, when I was finishing my meditation and I had completed my fast, I groped around until I found the stone. I held it up and I could not even see it. And I held it there and I prayed, 'My Father, my God, on this morning of the twenty-first day, I pray you will show me the light.' And I threw the stone away."

As he cast the stone aside, over on the horizon, he saw a little bitty beam of light, which started moving towards him. As it moved, it came faster and faster and got larger and larger and it frightened him nearly to death. He jumped to his feet and turned to run. He was really afraid, thinking to himself, "If that hits me, it'll kill me!"

Then he caught himself. He swung around and shouted "NO! I have spent years in my search. I have just asked to be shown the light. I will not run away!" He placed his feet and braced himself, and said, "Father, if it kills me, I'll accept the light."

And he said that when he made that decision, this light simply burst upon him. It struck him in the middle of his forehead and knocked him to the ground, unconscious. And he told Dr. Hyashi that he believed at that moment he had died.

The next thing he knew, he saw bubbles…millions and millions of bubbles moving from the right to the left in every color of the rainbow: from the palest pink to the deepest cerise, from the palest green to the deepest emerald, the palest aqua to the deepest blue. And after all these gorgeous colors, the gold and the white lights came.

In the center of every white bubble was a gold figure in the Sanskrit that he had learned and read in the sutras. The bubble would come and stop, as though to say, "Here Dr. Usui, learn this so you will know it and always be able to use it." And then it would go. And another would come in it's place. He was so afraid that he'd miss something, he told Dr. Hayashi, he didn't even blink!

Finally, he felt he had it all, and said, "Thank you, God. Now I have it. I know I can use it. Thank you, thank you, thank you."

The next thing he knew, he opened his eyes and it was broad daylight! It was the middle of the morning. He thought, "Ahhhhh! What a fantastic experience!"

He got to his feet, and decided, "I'll go back down the mountain and tell the bishop about this wonderful thing. I hope I am strong enough." And he started beating the dust off his shoes, flicked the pine needles and the dirt off his robe, put his hat on, grasped his staff, and thought, "It's a miracle! I have fasted for 21 days and I am strong! I can go all the way to Kyoto without any problem. It truly is a miracle."

He got so excited, he took off running down the mountainside, stubbed his toe on a rock, and tore his toenail clear back. And he did what all of us would have done. He sat right down and grabbed it and said "Ouch!" He held it with both hands. And he thought, "Ah, that feels very strange. I'll keep holding it until it quits hurting." Which it did. When he took his hands away, it was completely healed. And he thought to himself, "Ah! That's the second miracle!"

As he progressed on down the mountainside, he came to a bench with a red blanket on it with an ashtray in the middle. (And to this very day up in the mountains in Japan, that symbolizes fast food service—a Japanese McDonalds, so to speak.) He thought he'd stop and have some breakfast. And while the man was preparing him breakfast, his little daughter came out of the small hutch that they lived in.

She looked like a little cartoon character. She had a rag tied around her head, with a big knotty thing on top and one side of her face all pushed out. She was crying and crying. Dr. Usui said to her, "My dear child, what is the matter?"

She cried, "Oh good monk, I have this terrible toothache, and we live too far from Kyoto, so I can't go there. We're too poor to pay a dentist, and it just hurts so bad!"

He told her, "Come and sit here before me and let's see if I can help you." As she kneeled before him, he put his hands upon her, with one hand on the side of her swollen face.

She exclaimed, "Oh sir, you are not an ordinary monk."

"Why do you sat that child?" he asked.

She said, "Oh your hands are so hot!" After a few more minutes, she said, "Oh! You make magic. My tooth has stopped hurting!"

He said, "Isn't that wonderful? That's the third miracle."

After that he had his breakfast—and that was the fourth miracle. After fasting for 21 days, he was able to eat all those wonderful things that the Japanese think make a fine breakfast—raw fish and pickled plums and all those delicious treats! Believe me THAT was a miracle!

He proceeded down to Kyoto, and when he got to the door of the monastery and knocked on the door, the little boy came to the door and said, "Oh, Usui Sensei! I'm so glad to see you! I had all my friends together and we were coming out first thing in the morning for your bones!"

Dr. Usui said, "Thank you very much. As you see, that won't be necessary now. Where is the bishop?"

The little boy answered, "Oh, I have sad news, such sad, sad news."

"What's the matter?" asked Dr. Usui.

"The bishop is in his little room with his feet on a hibachi, all wrapped up in his blanket because his arthritis is nearly killing him."

"Oh I'm sorry to hear that. I will have something to eat and get a bath, and then I will go tell him about the wonderful things which have happened to me." Which he did.

With the bishop's permission, Dr. Usui sat with one hand on the bishop's hip and one hand on his back where his arthritis grew. Meanwhile, he talked about the wonderful experience he had. And after he had been talking to the man for a few minutes, the bishop turned to Dr. Usui and said, "Dr. Usui, you made magic!"

Usui inquired, "What's happening?"

The bishop exclaimed, "My arthritis has stopped hurting me!"

Dr. Usui said, "Isn't that wonderful. That is the Reiki. That's the Reiki that has been lost for so long!"

"Now how am I best going to use it?" he wondered aloud.

And the bishop suggested, "Well, I think we should meditate and pray a lot." And Dr. Usui agreed, so, they each went to their own room and spent the night in meditation and prayer.

Later, Dr Usui began working in a beggar camp in Japan, healing the sick. After seven years, when he saw beggars returning to the beggar camp, he realized that he had healed the physical body of symptoms, but he had not taught appreciation for life or a new way of living. He left the beggar camp to seek answers about how to heal body, mind, spirit, and emotions. Over many years, he perfected and refined the healing method, and he began teaching classes on Reiki.

One of his students, Dr. Chujiro Hayashi, was a retired Naval officer who became very involved in the practice of Reiki. When Dr. Usui's life was near its end, he recognized Dr. Hayashi as the

Master of Reiki and gave him the mandate to keep the essence and purity of his teachings.

Dr. Hayashi founded a clinic in Toyoko and kept careful records of healings. His records showed that Reiki finds the source of the physical symptoms, fills the vibration or energy need, and restores the body to wholeness.

Mrs. Takata was born on December 24, 1900, in Hawaii to two sugar cane workers of Japanese descent and culture. Her mother instructed the midwife, "Take the infant out into the sunrise. Name this child Hawayo after the big island. Then her name will be important, and she will become a worthy person." Decades later, that prophesy would be fulfilled.

Hawayo's formal education ended at the second grade. She then trained to be the house servant for an accountant at one of Hawaii's plantations, Saichi Takata. He fell in love with Hawayo and he married her. Mrs. Takata's life seemed established and secure in the Oriental tradition. She had a loving husband and two daughters to nurture. But it was not to last. At age of 31, Mrs. Takata was widowed.

Responsibility to care for not only her growing children but her parents too, fell upon her frail shoulders. As the stress began take a toll on her health, she became ill with a lung condition and also needed gallbladder surgery. Always hesitant to trust anyone she didn't know, Mrs. Takata faced the dilemma of knowing physicians only in the Tokyo clinic where her husband had once been a patient. She decided that is where she must go, the hardships of a long trip notwithstanding.

When Mrs. Takata's saved pennies totaled $50, she and her daughters booked passage on a cattle boat to Tokyo. Not surprisingly, she was too weak upon arrival at the clinic to undergo surgery. For six months, the Takata family lived at the clinic until she was strong enough for the operation. Then a strange thing happened.

On the morning of her surgery, as Mrs. Takata lay on the operating table while doctors scrubbed and nurses bustled about, she heard a voice mysteriously speak to her, "There's another way."

She looked around, seeing no one who could be talking to her. "I'm losing my mind," she whispered to herself. "I am hearing strange voices."

Just as she convinced herself it was her imagination, it came again: "There's another way."."

She tried to persuade herself that she was sleeping or anesthetized, before finally admitting to herself that she was fully conscious, as the voice came a third time, "There's another way!"

"Then what am I to do?" she asked mentally.

"Ask the doctor," replied the voice.

Taking a stance uncharacteristic for a woman raised in the Japanese tradition, Mrs. Takata faced her doctor and declared bluntly, "I think there's another way. There must be a better way. Is there any other kind of therapy or treatment that I can receive and try that you think will help me?"

The doctor, taken aback by this shocking challenge from the petite woman on whom he was about to begin surgery, recovered his composure and thought for a few moments.

"Yes." he answered. "How long can you remain in this country?"

"I can stay two years," something prompted Mrs. Takata to say.

"Wonderful," replied the surgeon. "If you have two years, wonderful. There is a better way!"

He turned to a nurse, instructing her to telephone his sister in the clinic's kitchen. His sister's ailment had been cured by another physician in Tokyo, one who administered drugless and bloodless treatments.

"Take Mrs. Takata to Shimano Machi," he told his sister without hesitation. Now, after more than three decades, the long-ago prophecy made by Hawayo Takata's mother was unfolding.

Enroute to the clinic where Machi worked, Mrs. Takata's guide eagerly spoke about her own physical healing there as they rode among Tokyo's maze of streets in a cab. Soon after, they arrived at the eight-bed clinic and met with some of its sixteen Reiki practitioners, all managed by Dr. Chujiro Hayashi, Dr. Usui's successor.

Any lingering doubts Mrs. Takata had quickly dissolved because she felt such welcoming warmth of Dr. Hayashi's smile and the hospitality of Mrs. Hayashi. "Yes," he assured Mrs. Takata, "I can help you."

Mrs. Takata described her first treatment. She said she felt so much electrical charge that she jumped up and looked under the sleeve of the kimono to see if there was something causing the vibrations and heat she felt. Once convinced of the Reiki energy, Mrs. Takata committed to study Reiki and her health began returning, as she continued treatments under the hands of Dr. Hayashi and his staff.

As mentioned earlier, right before Dr. Hayashi passed, he authorized Mrs. Takata as the guardian and Grand Master of Reiki. Upon Mrs. Takata's death, her granddaughter Phyllis Furumoto became the Grand Master. Phyllis founded the Reiki Alliance to protect and preserve the purity of the Reiki energy and its transmission as an oral tradition.

◆ ◆ ◆

ABOUT THE AUTHOR

ELEANOR HASPEL-PORTNER, PH.D.

Eleanor Haspel-Portner, Ph.D. became involved in meditation and energy work in the early 1970's. Reiki came to her attention in 1977 when she enrolled in a Reiki class to determine if it had any validity. Mrs. Takata was present at the Reiki class. After the first attunement Eleanor was instructed to go home that night and to work on herself using the four Reiki Head Positions. She followed the instructions and when she awoke the next morning, she noted that she could see without her glasses, which she wears for very severe myopia.

Something extraordinary had happened. Eleanor took this experience to mean that indeed there was validity to Reiki. After receiving the Second Reiki attunement, Eleanor noted that her perfect vision lasted for an even longer period of time. She received all First Degree Reiki initiations and went on to study Second Degree Reiki. At that time, Mrs. Takata did not make Third Degree Reiki available. Mrs. Takata passed the Reiki keys to others before her death in 1980, after which Reiki became more generally available. Eleanor studied Third Degree Reiki in 1981, and she is the tenth Reiki Master/Teacher initiated.

Eleanor received her Ph.D. from The University of Chicago, Department on Comparative Human Development, the first doctoral social science interdisciplinary department in the United States. Eleanor is a licensed clinical psychologist and professional certified coach. She uniquely integrates her background and training in psychology, biology, anthropology, and sociology with esoteric studies. She is a past president of the Southern California Society for Clinical Hypnosis, a certified ASCH approved consultant, certified Clean Language coach, and a member of numerous professional associations.

By applying multidimensional Noble Sciences Tools™ that she developed and validated, Eleanor helps people transform their lives. She helps thousands of individuals, couples, and groups synthesize their life experiences in practical ways for living healthy, successful, and creative lives. Eleanor strongly believes that each individual's core Self manifests fully when given support and encouragement. She also believes that many people simply need some directional help to feel empowered in their lives.

Eleanor and Marvin work together in documenting their work. They are both Tai Chi Gung teachers certified by the 3,300-year-old Lamasery in Tibet. They met in India on August 13, 1978, and continue to live closely together with furry loved ones. They hold a weekly FREE Manifest Your Dream Webinar (nobleenergywellness.com/free-webinar/). They enjoy their dogs and cats, and they love spending time with their children and grandchildren.

◆ ◆ ◆

COLLABORATIVE ASSISTANCE

MARVIN M. PORTNER, Ph.D.

Marvin Portner, M.D. had been doing healing work for many years when Eleanor introduced him to Reiki in 1978. The purity and the healing power of Reiki energy impressed him. Marvin found that the intensity and reliability of the energy work he did after his Reiki initiations brought a new dimension to his other work with patients. He expanded his study of Reiki through the years and has been consistently using and teaching it since he and Eleanor were initiated as Reiki Master Teachers in 1982.

Marvin M. Portner, M.D., was born in Detroit, Michigan on March 15. He is Board Certified in internal medicine, allergy, and immunology, both pediatric and adult. Marvin graduated from the University of Michigan Medical School with high honors. Although Marvin worked in traditional medicine for many years, he became an early pioneer in the field of holistic integratted medicine. He has been involved in synthesizing/integrating Western and Eastern medicine as well as working with mind/body medicine for over thirty-five years. His medical practice remains personalized and interactive, making him a rare practitioner in today's marketplace. Marvin practices as a medical consultant. He holds medical licenses in both California and in South Carolina.

CINDY SMITH

Cindy Smith was introduced to First and Second Degree Reiki by Eleanor, and in 2008 initiated as a Reiki Master by Eleanor and Marvin. Upon learning Reiki, Cindy began working with the Noble Energy Wellness tools and found them profoundly expansive in her own development. She and Eleanor worked together to develop Reiki Mind Maps that serve as a highly instructive tool in learning and using the tools taught in all levels of Reiki. Cindy is an avid student of philosophy and mysticism. She began working intensively with Noble Sciences™ tools and collaborates with Eleanor in further developing her materials. Cindy met her husband through a mutual love of skydiving. They have been married for 35 years and have one child. Cindy has a Master of Science in Information Systems and Technology Management.

Important Note

Through the years, many factions developed in the Reiki organization and individuals began to change the attunements and the teaching, thus diluting its energy and dissipating its integrity. Not all individuals who claim to teach Reiki have the keys to do the attunements, and some people who claim to teach Reiki do not even realize that a specific attunement process is required to set the energy path. Eleanor, Marvin, and Cindy continue to honor the purity of the Usui Reiki teaching and do the Usui Reiki attunements without any modifications to the system.

Noble Energy Wellness™

Noble Energy Wellness focuses on energy medicine and holistic options for healing and health. Dr. Marvin and Dr. Eleanor teach energy wellness in their weekly Manifest Your Dreams Webinar. Through the webinar, you can learn how to live authentically while manifesting your actual potential by understanding and integrating the Four Worlds into your daily life. Register to learn how you can manifest your dreams by attending these weekly webinars. https://nobleenergywellness.com

Noble Energy Maps™

Noble Energy Maps focus on Dr. Eleanor's proprietary and innovative system for mapping how cosmic energy impacted you during your childhood development and how you can use this knowledge to optimally time your decisions, identify your life purpose, and live a self-realized life. Dr. Eleanor statistically validated her system through over 45,000 cases and uses Noble Energy Maps to guide clients toward wholeness and empowerment. https://www.nobleenergywellness.com/energy-map/

The Noble logo has a special place in Dr. Eleanor's heart. Her first cat, Noble, lived to age 22 and was an inspiration and guide during important times in Dr. Eleanor's growth and studies. He worked with her and Dr. Marvin when they hosted weekend groups for over ten years. Noble always helped guide them toward whom to work with next, as well as to the area

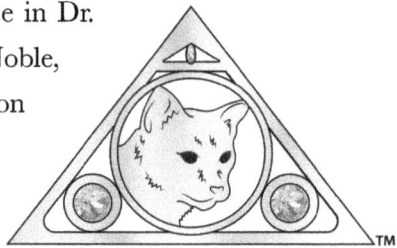

that clients needed to work on. Dr. Eleanor uses calculations based on research done on her two homegrown twin kittens. The critical human developmental times used in Dr. Eleanor's proprietary maps, have proven accurate clinically and statistically, which map the Four Worlds in your energy field and how you can best function.

The Mandala of Synthesis describes the elements coded into Dr. Eleanor's proprietary Noble Energy Maps. The Mandala of Synthesis includes the Kabbalistic Tree of Life, Chakras, Astrology, the Hexagrams of the I-Ching, and critical times in early human development. Dr. Eleanor calculates her maps and integrates the information coded into a graphic

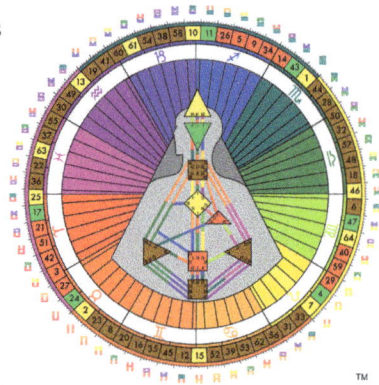

illustrating the way you use your energy, where the flow of energy becomes clear. Dr. Eleanor's extensive education as a social scientist, researcher, and clinician has empowered her to formulate a complete system that recognizes the complexity of your consciousness and shows how you can best use it for growth and expansion of consciousness.

https://www.nobleenergywellness.com/mandala-of-synthesis